Ketogenic Diet Recipes:

The Fundamental Guide to High Fat, Low-Carb for Ketogenic Diet Beginners.

Table of Contents

Introduction

PUT QUITE SIMPLY, the Ketogenic diet is a high-fat, low carb, moderate protein diet. Got it? Great. Now let's get into the specifics. It is really quite simple. Once you get started on it, you'll find it to be very intuitive.

All human bodies require three main macronutrients to survive: carbohydrates, proteins, and fats. For years, we have been taught that we need to eat a high carb, moderate protein, and low fat diet. But what has that really lead to? High rates of obesity, sickness, and poor health across the board. Eating high carb leads people to go on binges, eating too much, and making themselves sick. What if we change our thinking, and entirely change the focus of our diets?

The Keto diet changes the focus from carbs to fat. On a Keto diet, you want your intake to be very high-fat, with close to zero carbohydrates. Most Keto practitioners eat 80% of their daily calories from fat. So what does that look like?

1 gram of fat has 9 calories. So if you're operating on a 2,000-calorie diet per day, you need 80% of that to come from fat. 80% of 2,000 calories would be 1,600 calories, or 178 grams of fat per day. Don't

worry, there isn't this much math involved in day-to-day Keto eating!

Okay, but what about the other two macronutrients? On a Keto diet, you'll eat 80% fat, 15% protein, and only 5% carbs. Let's continue with our 2,000-calorie example. 1 gram of carbohydrates and protein both have 4 calories. On a 2,000-calorie diet, you'll want 15% to be protein, which works out to 300 calories, or 75 grams of protein. Carbs are even less — 5% of your 2,000 calories. That ends up being only 100 calories, or 25 grams of carbohydrates.

So in a typical Keto day, you'll eat 178 grams of fat, 75 grams of protein, and 25 grams of carbohydrates. If you're feeling a bit overwhelmed, don't worry, we're going to do the hard work for you. At the end of this book, we've included a meal plan and list of meal suggestions so you can easily stay within these guidelines.

The big takeaway is this: on Keto, you get almost all of your daily calories from fats, and reduce your intake of carbohydrates down close to nothing.

Part one: What is Ketogenic Diet

Ketogenic dieting is a very simple and effective way to lose weight. Ketogenic dieting has two main objectives. It focuses on limiting carbohydrate intake in order to burn excess body fat first and foremost. Secondly, it also focuses on increasing fat intake to replace the energy lost as a result of the removal of carbohydrates from your diet. This makes for a pretty simple diet plan right? It frees you from counting calories or eating six meals a day, or what ever the newest fad diets are saying nowadays. Simply avoid carbohydrates and eat more fat. Any one can do that.

By removing carbohydrates from your diet your body will naturally go in to a state of ketosis. During ketosis your body adapts to burning fat for energy. This is the secret to burning pounds of fat quickly and effortlessly. This is why low carbohydrate dieting has become so popular in the last decade. People actually see results when they cut out carbohydrates, but still get to eat as much as they want.

How our bodies get energy

There are three major forms of energy that our bodies use as fuel. The first and most readily available are carbohydrates. Carbohydrates are made up of sugars and starches which are easily accessed for energy the body may need. The second source of energy the body uses is from fats. These can come from plants or animals and are less easily used for energy, but also make up the energy reserves that our bodies store around our middle section for later use. The third source of energy that our bodies can use is protein. This is the least desirable source of energy as it is the most difficult to access and will reduce muscle mass in times of starvation.

Our bodies are accustomed to using carbohydrates as our number one source of energy. This makes it very difficult for many people to lose weight. No matter how much they cut calories or exercise, their bodies just don't respond to the diet by losing weight. Part of the problem is that when carbohydrates are the body's normal source of energy it keeps insulin levels in the blood high.

The body uses insulin as a gatekeeper to allow sugars from carbohydrates into cells for fuel. As more carbohydrates are consumed, more insulin is produced to allow the cells to utilize the sugar. The problem with insulin in the blood constantly, besides being the predominant cause of type II diabetes, is that is inhibits the ability of the body to breakdown fat for energy. So no matter how many calories you cut out of your diet, your body is working against you to lose fat if you are eating carbohydrates consistently.

This can be especially confounding when our bodies go in to adaptive thermogenesis, or "starvation mode", from reduced calories. Adaptive thermogenesis can result in hundreds of fewer calories burned a day when dieting. So with the typical calorie restriction diet you must overcome the body's resistance to breaking down fat cells due to increased insulin levels from carbohydrates and the adaptive thermogenesis that will occur from reduced calories. It is no wonder so many people cannot succeed with traditional dieting. It is not their fault, it is all of the new diets that come out reduce fat intake and calories.

Ketogenic dieting changes how the body gets energy

So if you go out for a nice steak dinner and you eat a juicy steak, but you also eat bread and some sort of potato on the side, your body is going to find its energy in the potato and bread and ignore the fat from the steak. The problem is that there is so much extra energy in the bread and potato that it will get stored as fat as an evolutionary precaution against famine. You body bypasses the fat energy from the steak and the cycle continues at the next meal so that you never dip in to your fat reserves.

This is where the ketogenic diet changes things. When you significantly reduce the amount of carbohydrates your body takes in, you change where your body gets it's energy from. It no longer looks for this energy from carbohydrates, but from fat. When the body runs out of sugars that it has stored in the liver it uses ketones to start fueling all of its processes. This is when ketogenesis begins. Ketogenesis is when dietary fats are turned in to ketones for energy. When the body uses these ketones as energy it has entered a state of ketosis. That is the goal of ketogenic dieting because it trains the body to use its fat stores instead of holding out for more sugar when it needs energy. That is the reason people see such dramatic fat loss results while ketogenic dieting.

History of ketogenic dieting

 The ketogenic diet is not some new fad diet. I has been around for quite a while in fact. The history of ketogenic dieting may surprise you, though. It was popularized in the 1920's to help fight against epilepsy. In the early 20th century there were few good options for treating epilepsy and many people resorted to fasting as an alternative treatment. Fasting had been know as a treatment for epilepsy for over 1,500 years at that point but was difficult to follow strictly. A study published in 1916 in the New York Medical Journal found that 70% of patients who adhered to a fast diet improved in some way. A full 20% of the participants had no symptoms at all while on the fast diet.

The difficulty of adhering to a fast diet lead some to look for alternatives to this method. In 1921 an endocrinologist named Rollin Woodatt found that three water soluble compounds; acetone, β-hydroxybutyrate and acetoacetate, which together are called ketone bodies, were produced by the liver as a result of starvation or by following a diet rich in fat and low in carbohydrates. That same year Russel Wilder from the Mayo clinic began using this form of dieting to treat epilepsy, calling the ketogenic diet.

Since then the ketogenic diet has been used as an alternative treatment for epilepsy and is currently being studied for its positive effects on other neurological diseases as well. It gained popularity as a means of fat loss much more recently and has many people turning to it as a lifestyle change that not only promotes good health, but also actually has results in significant fat loss. Undoubtedly the ketogenic diet will have its place as a tool for fat loss and health optimization as well as an alternative treatment for many health issues for a long time to come. As new research emerges touting its effectiveness, it will become more and more popular.

Part two: 7 day diet meal plan

Now you have all the knowledge needed for the Ketogenic diet, it's time to kick-start your weight loss with this 7-day Keto meal plan!

Our main goal here is to stay simple as simplicity is key for someone that is just starting out on a keto diet.

In this section, you will find weekly meal plans with breakfast, lunch, snack and dinner.

Weekday Breakfast

For breakfast, you want something that's quick and easy, and of course, tasty. Therefore, most of the weekday breakfasts will simply be shakes, bacon or sausage and eggs, or bulletproof coffee as they are easy to make and can provide you with the high fat you need first thing in the morning. This is to keep things simple so you can stick to the plan.

Weekday Lunch

For lunch, we will also keep it simple. Most of the time, it will be salad, meat or something that's easy to be put into a container and bring to work.

Weekday Snack

The key to success in this 30-day keto meal plan is that you don't get hungry. Therefore, I highly suggest that you bring some snacks with you everyday to get you through the cravings. It can be as easy as pork rinds, beef jerky or fat bombs. Just remember to always be prepared so you don't go crazy and end up eating things you're not supposed to have.

Weekday Dinner

Dinner will be something that is high on the fat and moderate on the protein. Most of them are quick and easy to prepare. Just make sure to cook ahead if it's a slow cooker recipe.

Weekend Meals

After a busy week, it is time to give yourself a treat. You will see in the meal plan that on the 6th and 7th days (Saturday and Sunday), we usually will have something a little special that will satisfy your cravings.

How to Use the 7-day Meal Plan

•	Check the weekly meal plan and recipes beforehand and have all your ingredients prepared.

•	Customize the meal plan: if there are recipes or certain ingredients you don't like, feel free to replace them by other recipes or ingredients that are keto-friendly.

•	For weekday lunches and snacks, make them the night and store them in the containers before so you can just grab them when you go to work. You may also consider one or two meal prepping sections during the week. You can even pack dinner leftovers as lunch the following day.

WEEK ONE MEAL PLAN

DAY 1 (MONDAY)

•	Breakfast: Avocado Coconut Milk Shake

•	Lunch: Avocado Caesar Salad

- Snack: Mixed Roasted Nuts

- Dinner: Chicken Broccoli Stir-Fry

Day 2 (Tuesday)

- Breakfast: Cinnamon Chia Pudding

- Lunch: Grilled Salmon & Asparagus

- Snack: Pork rinds

- Dinner: Cauliflower Mac & Cheese

Day 3 (Wednesday)

- Breakfast: Avocado, Ham and Egg

- Lunch: Thai Zoodles (Pad Thai)

- Snack: Dark chocolate

- Dinner: Spaghetti Squash Burrito Bowls

Day 4 (Thursday)

- Breakfast: Bulletproof coffee

- Lunch: Taco salad

- Snack: Parmesan Chips

- Dinner: Dijon Mustard Chicken with vegetables

Day 5 (Friday)

- Breakfast: Bacon and eggs

- Lunch: Cauliflower rice + Mustard Chicken and vegetables (Leftover from the night before)

- Snack: Parmesan Chips

- Dinner: Lettuce Wrap Cheeseburger

Day 6 (Saturday)

- Breakfast: Keto Cream Cheese Pancake

- Lunch: Sausage Casserole

- Snack: Easy Keto Vanilla Ice Cream

- Dinner: Crockpot Beef Stew

Day 7 (Sunday)

- Breakfast: Bulletproof coffee

- Lunch: Oven Roasted Brussels Sprouts with Bacon and Cheese

- Snack: Easy Keto Vanilla Ice Cream

- Dinner: Baked Buffalo Chicken Tender

Benefits of the Ketogenic Diet

There are a number of benefits to the ketogenic diet including reduced appetite, increased weight loss, reduced triglycerides, reduced cholesterol and more! In this chapter we are going to take a look at these benefits and examine why they occur in the ketogenic diet.

The Ketogenic Diet Causes a Reduction in Appetite

Perhaps one of the biggest downsides to any diet is the feeling of constant hunger. Very often this hunger then leads to binging, and of course this is almost always acted upon with unhealthy foods. The ketogenic diet helps to reduce this type of sabotage because it reduces the appetite. How does this happen? When a diet includes fewer carbohydrates and a higher quantity of fats the body actually feels a greater level of satisfaction than it would if it were simply consuming more carbohydrates. Additionally, when the body experiences the release of ketone bodies, the appetite is reduced.

No Sudden Drops in Blood Sugar

Due to the fact that during ketosis the body is feeding on fats rather than carbohydrates, glucose levels are lower and more static. This means that you will no longer experience those significant drops (or spikes) in blood sugar that come with eating carbohydrate heavy foods!

Reduced Blood Pressure

Research shows that a reduction in carbohydrates is directly linked to a reduction in blood pressure. Consequently, the ketogenic diet has the effect of lowering the blood pressure. With high blood pressure linked to a number of health conditions including strokes and heart disease, lowering blood pressure is a great benefit to this eating plan!

Increased HDL Levels

HDL, also known as "good cholesterol" which takes cholesterol from the body to the liver for excretion or use, has been shown to increase dramatically when eating a low carbohydrate diet that focuses on higher fat consumption. As with high blood pressure, high cholesterol is linked to a number of health conditions, so increasing good cholesterol levels is very beneficial.

Increased Weight Loss

Increased weight loss is a direct result of the ketogenic diet for a lot of the reasons. In addition, the ketogenic involves eating more fats and proteins which tend to lead to consuming fewer calories per sitting when compared to eating carbohydrate rich diets.

Reduced Triglycerides

Increased levels of triglycerides have been directly linked to heart health. Just as detrimental as high cholesterol, it is important for heart health to bring down high triglyceride levels and this can be done through the ketogenic diet. The most significant culprit for causing high levels of triglycerides is the consumption of carbohydrates, so significantly reducing carbs directly reduces triglycerides.

Reduced Cholesterol

In addition to increasing HDL cholesterol levels, the ketogenic diet also reduces LDL cholesterol. High levels of LDL cholesterol, or "bad cholesterol" are directly linked to the risk of heart attack. The ketogenic diet helps to reduce these levels of LDL cholesterol by enlarging the present LDL particles in the blood so that there are less of them present.

Reduced "Belly Fat"

Visceral fat, or the fat that is found in the abdomen. This type of fat tends to lead to health conditions because it has a habit of collecting around the body's organs. The ketogenic diet has been proven to reduce abdominal fat as well as increase the average level of fat lost in the dieter.

Reduced Insulin Levels

Due to the fact that there is a lack of carbohydrates, and consequently glucose in the body, the levels of insulin are also decreased.

Reduced Pain and Stiffness in the Joints

Many people suffer from swelling and pain as a result of having grains present in their diet. The ketogenic diet eliminates these grains, thereby significantly reducing a lot of joint stiffness and muscle tension.

Improved Mental Health

The ketone bodies that are released when adhering to the ketogenic diet have been directly linked to mental health. Studies have shown that increased ketone levels lead to stabilization of neurotransmitters like dopamine and serotonin. This stabilization can help to combat depression as well as lead to less mood swings.

Improved Digestion

Eating a diet like the ketogenic diet, that is low in grains and sugars, results in an incredible improvement in digestion. Consumption of both sugars and grains has been shown to result in gas, bloating, stomach pains and even constipation. Eliminating or drastically reducing sugars and carbohydrates decreases, and in most case eliminates, these digestive symptoms.

1.   Breakfast

One Pan Breakfast

(Prep Time: 15 MIN| Serve: 4)

Ingredients

- 8 slices bacon
- 4 pcs. free-range eggs
- 1 medium-sized carrots julienned
- ½ cup celery, chopped
- ½ cup cauliflower, chopped
- 1 small white onion, chopped
- ½ cup gouda cheese, shredded
- 1 tbsp. butter

Directions

1. Prepare the vegetables and bacon.
2. Heat a large pan over medium fire and add the 1 tbsp. butter to melt.
3. Throw in the chopped vegetables and bacon and sauté for 20 mins or until the bacon is almost crisp. Remember to stir often.

4.   Using a spatula, spread the vegetables and bacon evenly on the pan and then create four well.
5.   Take one egg and then break it into the well. Do the same for the rest of the eggs.
6.   Cover the pan with a lid and then heat until the eggs are cooked to your liking.
7.   Turn off the heat and then sprinkle with the shredded cheese. Serve.

Nutritional Values

- Calories: 385 kcal

- Fat: 33.05g

- Carbohydrates: 5.58g

- Protein: 16.19g

- Dietary Fiber: 1.2g

- Cholesterol: 629mg

All-In Omelet

(Prep Time: 5 MIN| Serve: 2)

Ingredients

- 4 eggs whites from a free range egg
- 1 pc. yolk
- 1 pc. heirloom tomato, chopped
- 1 cup baby spinach, roughly chopped
- ¼ cup cheddar, shredded
- 1 small white onion, chopped
- ½ tsp. dried basil
- 2 tbsp. coconut milk
- 1 tbsp. butter

Directions

1. Place all the egg whites and yolk in a mixing bowl. Add the 2 tbsp. coconut milk and whisk all the ingredients together.
2. Melt the butter on a non-stick pan over medium fire. Throw in the baby spinach, cheddar, chopped tomato, and onion. Sauté for 5 minutes or until the spinach is wilted. Set aside.
3. Transfer the sautéed vegetables on a plate and set aside.

4.   Pour the egg mixture into the same pan and cook the eggs until done.

5.   Place the cooked egg on a serving plate and then top one half of the egg with the cooked vegetables. Fold the egg and to create an omelet. Serve.

Nutritional Values

- Calories: 601 kcal

- Fat: 33.57g

- Carbohydrates: 8.95g

- Protein: 25.29g

- Dietary Fiber : 1.5g

- Cholesterol: 1363mg

Heavenly Cakes

(Prep Time: 20 MIN| Serve: 3)

Ingredients

- 6 free-range eggs
- 350 grams ham, cooked and cut into cubes
- 1 yellow onion, chopped
- 2 tbsp. onion chopped chives
- 1 cup shredded cheddar
- 3 tbsp. plus 1 tbsp. butter
- ½ cup heavy cream

Directions

1. Preheat the oven at 400F.
2. Melt the 3 tbsp. butter in a skillet heated over medium fire.
3. Add the onions to the pan and sauté until the onions are translucent. Add the garlic and sauté for another minute or two. Turn off the heat and transfer the in a large bowl.
4. Add the rest of the ingredients in the bowl with the sautéed vegetables except for the 1 tbsp. butter. Stir well and set aside.

5. Take 6 pcs. of ramekins and brush it with the 1 tbsp. butter. Pour the mixture into the prepared ramekins filling only ½ of the cups.

6. Place in the oven to cook for 20 minutes or until the top turns light brown. Serve.

Nutritional Values

- Calories: 420 kcal

- Fat: 31.87g

- Carbohydrates: 7.55g

- Protein: 25.52g

- Dietary Fiber : 0.7g

- Cholesterol: 1291mg

Pesto And Eggs

(Prep Time: 15 MIN| Serve: 3)

Ingredients

- 1 ½ tbsp. pesto sauce
- 4 free-range eggs
- 2 tbsp. butter
- 3 tbsp. source cream

Directions

1. Whisk the eggs in a bowl. You can lightly season it with salt and pepper.
2. Heat a non-stick pan over medium fire. Melt the butter and then pour the whisked egg on the hot pan.
3. Add the pesto sauce to the pan and stir.
4. Turn off the heat and then add the 3 scoops of sour cream. Stir well.
5. You can serve with on the side of a mashed avocado.

Nutritional Values

- Calories: 210 kcal

- Fat: 22.46g
- Carbohydrates: 1.31g
- Protein: 1.9g
- Dietary Fiber : 0.1g
- Cholesterol: 47mg

Ketogenic Pancakes

(Prep Time: 10 MIN| Serve: 2)

Ingredients

- 4 large free-range eggs
- ¾ cup nut butter
- ½ tsp. baking soda
- 1 tsp. cinnamon powder
- 1/3 cup coconut milk
- 2 tbsp. of a sugar substitute like stevia or erythritol
- 2 tbsp. butter or clarified butter

Directions

1. Add all the ingredients in a food processor (except the 2 tbsp. butter) and pulse until all the ingredients are thoroughly combined. Set aside.
2. Melt the butter on a non-stick pan over low fire. Scoop ¼ cup of the pancake batter into the hot pan and then cook until the pancake has set, flip and cook until finished.
3. Repeat the same procedure for the rest of the batter. You can serve this

with a drizzle of an all-natural maple
syrup.

Nutritional Values

- Calories: 329 kcal

- Fat: 29.11g

- Carbohydrates: 13.32g

- Protein: 7.39g

- Dietary Fiber : 1.4g

- Cholesterol: 161mg

Bread-Free Sandwich

(Prep Time: 8 MIN| Serve: 2)

Ingredients

- 4 large free-range eggs
- 2 slices of pre-cooked ham
- 4 tbsp. provolone cheese, cut into thick slices
- A dash of Sriracha sauce
- A pinch of salt and pepper to taste
- 1 tbsp. butter

Directions

1. Melt the butter on a non-stick pan over medium fire. Crack the eggs, season with salt and pepper and fry until over easy.
2. Sandwich the slices of ham and cheese in between 2 cooked eggs.
3. Add a dash of Sriracha for an added kick (optional) and serve.

Nutritional Values

- Calories: 253 kcal

- Fat: 17.96g
- Carbohydrates: 6.9g
- Protein: 15.99g
- Dietary Fiber : 0.3g
- Cholesterol: 399mg

Cheesy Sausage Pie

(Prep Time: 8 MIN| Serve: 4)

Ingredients

- ¾ cup plus 2 tbsp. cheddar cheese, grated
- 2 pcs. chicken sausages
- ¼ cup coconut flour
- ¼ tsp. baking soda
- ½ tsp rosemary
- ¼ tsp. cayenne
- A pinch of kosher salt
- 5 egg yolks (free range)
- ¼ cup coconut oil
- 2 tbsp. coconut milk
- 2 tsp. lime juice

Directions

1. Preheat oven at 350F.
2. Slice the chicken sausages into small chunks and place on a heated skillet greased with butter.
3. While waiting for the sausages to cook, combine the ¼ cup cheddar, coconut flour, baking soda, rosemary, cayenne, and salt in a mixing bowl.

4.   In a separate bowl, mix the yolks, coconut oil, coconut milk, and lime juice. Stir well.
5.   Gradually add the wet ingredients into the bowl with the dry ingredients and fold to incorporate all the ingredients together.
6.   Pour the mixture into 2 ramekins and add the cooked sausages also in the ramekins.
7.   Place in the oven to cook for 25 minutes or until the pies turn light brown.
8.   Add the remaining cheddar on top of the pies and place back in the oven to melt the cheese for 4-5 minutes. Serve.

Nutritional Values

- Calories: 613 kcal
- Fat: 55.06g
- Carbohydrates: 5.39g
- Protein: 24.84g
- Dietary Fiber : 0.4g
- Cholesterol: 1562mg

Egg And Avocado Salad

(Prep Time: 5 MIN| Serve: 2)

Ingredients

- 4 pcs. free range eggs
- 1 oc. avocado
- 1 tsp. Dijon mustard
- ¼ cup mayonnaise
- 2 tbsp. cream cheese
- 1 scallion, chopped
- A pinch of kosher salt and pepper to taste

Directions

1. Boil the eggs in a pot for 10 mins. When done, run the boiled eggs with tap water. Remove the peel and then chop.
2. In a mixing bowl, combine the chopped eggs, mustard, mayo, cream cheese, and scallion. Lightly season it salt and pepper.
3. Cut the avocado in half and scoop out the flesh. Discard the peel and pit and add the flesh into the egg salad. Serve.

Nutritional Values
- Calories: 382 kcal
- Fat: 31.99g
- Carbohydrates: 9.91g
- Protein: 16.65g
- Dietary Fiber : 5.1g
- Cholesterol: 834mg

2.   Snacks

Avocado Chocolate Pudding

(Prep Time: 10 MIN| Serve: 4)

Ingredients

- 1 tbsp. coconut milk
- 1 avocado
- 2½ tbsp. raw cocoa powder
- 1 pinch sea salt
- ½ tbsp. vanilla extract
- 1 tsp ceylon cinnamon
- 1 tbsp coconut sugar
- 1 pinch stevia
- 1/16 tsp ground cayenne pepper

Directions

1. Cut and pit the avocado into a blender.
2. Blend until smooth.
3. Add in the coconut milk, cocoa powder and vanilla extract. Blend until smooth.

4.   Add in coconut sugar, cayenne pepper, stevia and cinnamon.

5.   Continue blending and make sure that all the chunks are blended by scraping down the sides of the food processor.

6.   Serve with sprinkle of sea salt on the pudding.

Nutritional Values

- Calories: 180 kcal
- Fat: 15g (84.9%)
- Carbohydrates: 3.5g (7.6%)
- Protein: 3g (7.5%)

Crunchy Kale Chips

(Prep Time: 15 MIN| Serve: 4)

Ingredients

- 1 tsp soy sauce
- 1 tps fish sauce
- 2 tbsp sriracha
- 2 tbsp olive oil
- 1 bunch of kale
- 1tsp of sea salt

Directions

1. Remove the kale from the stems
2. Preheat oven to 350 F
3. Line with parchment paper
4. Break it into chip sized pieces and placed it in a bowl.
5. Add sriracha, olive oil, soy sauce and fish sauce.
6. Swirl the mixture and pour the dressing over the kale leaves.
7. Place the leaves out on the parchment paper
8. Baked until crisp. Approx. 8 – 12 minutes.

9.   Sprinkling the sea salt over the kale
        leaves
10.   Serve it.

Nutritional Values
*   Calories: 49 kcal
*   Fat: 0.9g
*   Carbohydrates: 9g
*   Protein: 4.3g
*   Dietary Fiber : 1g
*   Cholesterol: 0mg

Granola Bars

(Prep Time: 25 MIN| Serve: 4)

Ingredients

- 2 eggs
- 1 tbsp. nut butter
- 2 tsp dried cinnamon
- 2 tbsp. cocoa nibs
- 1 tsp vanilla
- 50g shredded coconut
- 100g almonds
- 50g pumpkin seeds
- 50g linseed
- 50g sunflower seeds
- 50g pumpkin seeds
- 50g macadamia nuts
- 3 tbsp. stevia
- 50g coconut oil

Directions

1. Mix all the ingredients into the blender
2. Blend until smooth but little chunks of nuts and seeds are still visible.
3. Form 10 bars and place it on a dish with lined parchment paper

4.   Bake at 350F until golden or for 20 minutes.

Nutritional Values

- Calories: 245 kcal
- Fat: 21g
- Carbohydrates: 7g
- Protein: 7g
- Dietary Fiber : 4.5g
- Cholesterol: 0mg

Pepper Sea Salt Pork Rinds

(Prep Time: 35 MIN| Serve: 3)

Ingredients

- Pinch sea salt
- Pepper
- 2 to 4 lbs pork back fat and skin
- coconut oil

Directions

1. Preheat oven to 250F
2. Slice the pork skin and fat into long strips carefully. A sharp knife is required.
3. Separate a portion of the fat from the skin from one end of the strip.
4. Slice further to remove remaining fat.
5. Cut each strip into squares.
6. Place the strip (fat-side) down, on the wire rack with a baking sheet beneath.
7. Bake until the skin is crisp. Approx. 3 hours.
8. Pour the coconut oil into the pan.
9. Heat up the oil.

10.	Add the pork rinds and cook until they puff up. Approx. 3 – 5 minutes.
11.	Drain on a paper towel-lined plate.
12.	Serve with sprinkle of pepper and sea salt.

Nutritional Values

- Calories: 152 kcal
- Fat: 20g (100%)
- Carbohydrates: 0g
- Protein: 0g
- Dietary Fiber : 1g
- Cholesterol: 0mg

Salted Crispy Macadamia Nuts

(Prep Time: 15 MIN| Serve: 4)

Ingredients

- 3lb raw macadamia nuts
- 3 tbsp. sea salt
- filtered water

Directions

1. Mix the nuts and sea salt in a bowl and cover by 3 inches of water
2. Leave the bowl in a warm area for 8 hours.
3. Drain the nuts, and put them back in the bowl.
4. Add another few teaspoons of sea salt to season.
5. Place the nuts in your oven on lowest setting until dried out.

Nutritional Values

- Calories: 945kcal
- Fat: 100g
- Carbohydrates: 17g
- Protein: 10g
- Dietary Fiber : 11g

- Cholesterol: omg

Hard Boiled Egg

(Prep Time: 10 MIN| Serve: 2)

Ingredients

- 4 eggs

Directions

1. Place the eggs into a pot.
2. Cover it with water with the eggs submerge.
3. Boil over medium-high heat
4. Place lid over the pot
5. Remove and let it cool for 10 minutes.
6. Serve it.

Nutritional Values

- Calories: 202 kcal
- Fat: 14g
- Carbohydrates: 2g
- Protein: 17g
- Dietary Fiber : 0g
- Cholesterol: 373mg

Cheesy Bacon Wrap Sticks

(Prep Time: 25 MIN| Serve: 3)

Ingredients

- 4 slices of bacon
- coconut oil
- 2 mozzarella cheese sticks
- 1 egg

Directions

1. Beat the egg in a bowl
2. Slice the cheese stick into quarters.
3. Preheat coconut oil in deep fryer to 350 F
4. Dip the ends of the bacon into the bowl.
5. Wrap the cheese sticks with bacon.
6. Drop the bacon wrapped cheese into the deep fryer
7. Cook until the bacon is brown and crispy. Approx. 2 – 3 minutes.
8. Transfer over to a plate with paper towel.
9. Serve it.

Nutritional Values
- Calories: 113 kcal
- Fat: 9g
- Carbohydrates: 1g
- Protein: 7g
- Dietary Fiber : 0g
- Cholesterol: 0 mg

Fried Avocado With Lemon

(Prep Time: 8 MIN| Serve: 2)

Ingredients

- 1 avocado
- 1 tbsp. lemon juice
- 1 tbsp. coconut oil
- pinch of sea salt

Directions

1. Remove the seed and slice the avocado into pieces
2. Preheat the pan with coconut oil
3. Fry the avocado slices till gentle brown.
4. Sprinkle the lemon juice and sea salt over the slices.
5. Serve it.

Nutritional Values

- Calories: 180 kcal
- Fat: 18g
- Carbohydrates: 9g
- Protein: 3g
- Dietary Fiber : 7g
- Cholesterol: 0mg

Keto Meatballs

(Prep Time: 25 MIN| Serve: 2)

Ingredients

- 500g ground beef
- 2 eggs
- 1 tsp dried tyme
- 1 tsp sea salt
- 2 cloves garlic, minced
- 1 tsp dried oregano
- coconut flour
- 1 cup diced mozzarella
- freshly grounded black pepper
- ½ cup coconut flour

Directions

1. Preheat the over to 450F
2. Dice the mozzarella in 20 -25 square pieces
3. Place it in freezer for 45 - 60 minutes
4. Combine all the ingredients into a large bowl.
5. Mix and Stir with your clean hands
6. Roll the meat into 20 – 25 pieces
7. Remove the cheese from freezer
8. Wrap the meat over the cheese.

9.   Roll between hands and placed it on the baking tray with parchment paper.
10.   Bake for 13 – 15 minutes.
11.   Serve it.

Nutritional Values

- Calories: 117kcal
- Fat: 9.3g
- Carbohydrates: 1.4g
- Protein: 7g
- Dietary Fiber : 0.5g
- Cholesterol: mg

3.   Fish

Easy Salmon Salad With Avocado

(Prep Time: 15 MIN| Serve: 2)

Ingredients

- 1 pc. salmon fillet
- 1 pc. green onion, chopped
- 2 tbsp. lime juice
- ¼ cup keto mayo
- 2 tbsp. fresh dill
- 1 tbsp. ghee
- 1 avocado
- Pinch of salt and pepper

Directions

1. Set oven at 400F.
2. Lay the salmon fillet on a baking sheet lined with parchment paper. Drizzle with juice of lime and ghee on top.
3. Season the salmon with salt and pepper and place in the oven to bake for 25 minutes.

4.   When cooked, pull the salmon meat using a fork and place in a bowl.
5.   Add the mayo and green onions in the bowl and stir.
6.   Mash the avocado and add to the salmon salad. Lightly toss the ingredients together and serve.

Nutritional Values
- Calories: 490 kcal
- Fat: 31.99g
- Carbohydrates: 30.21g
- Protein: 26.7g
- Dietary Fiber : 9.3g
- Cholesterol: 94mg

Salmon Fillets

(Prep Time: 25 MIN| Serve: 3)

Ingredients

- 1 lb. salmon fillet
- ¼ cup button mushrooms, chopped
- 1 clove of garlic, minced
- ½ cup scallions, chopped
- ¼ cup tamari
- ¼ tsp. rosemary
- ¼ tsp. thyme
- ¼ tsp. tarragon
- ¼ tsp. basil
- ¼ tsp. oregano
- ¼ tsp. ginger, ground
- 2 tbsp. butter

Directions

1. Set oven at 350F.
2. Place the fish fillet in a re-sealable plastic bag and pour over the tamari, coconut oil, as well as the herbs and spices. Shake the bag well to coat the fish with the sauce and marinate in the fridge for 4 hours.

3.   When done marinating, place the salmon fillet on a baking sheet lined with foil and bake for at least 10 minutes.
4.   Melt the butter on a pan over medium heat. Add the mushrooms and scallions into the pan and cook until tender.
5.   Take the salmon out from the oven and pour over the sautéed mushrooms. Place the fish back in the oven to bake for another 10 mins. Serve.

Nutritional Values
- Calories: 323 kcal
- Fat: 18.62g
- Carbohydrates: 3.35g
- Protein: 34.46g
- Dietary Fiber : 0.8g
- Cholesterol: 122mg

Parmesan Crusted Fish

(Prep Time: 25 MIN| Serve: 2)

Ingredients

- 1 lb. cream dory fillet
- 2 tbsp. milk
- 1 egg
- ¼ cup parmesan cheese, grated
- 2 tbsp. almond flour
- ½ tsp. smoked paprika
- Pinch of salt and pepper to taste

Directions

1. Set the oven at 350F
2. Whisk the egg and milk together in a bowl.
3. In a re-sealable plastic bag combine all the dry ingredients and shake well.
4. Dip the fish fillet into the egg and milk mixture and place inside the plastic bag. Shake to cover the fillets with the breading.

5.	Place the fish fillets on a baking sheet lined with foil and cook in the oven for 25 minutes.
6.	Serve with lemon wedges on the side.

Nutritional Values
*	Calories: 293 kcal
*	Fat: 26.65g
*	Carbohydrates: 6.99g
*	Protein: 7.71g
*	Dietary Fiber : 0.3g
*	Cholesterol: 236mg

Fish In Orange Pecan Butter Sauce

(Prep Time: 35 MIN| Serve: 2)

Ingredients

- 1 pc. trout fillet, skin on
- ½ cup pecan nuts, chopped
- 1 pc. orange, juiced and zested
- 2 tbsp. butter, divided
- 1 tbsp. parsley, chopped
- A pinch of salt and pepper to taste

Directions

1. Melt 1 tbsp. of butter on a cast iron skillet over medium fire.
2. Flavor the trout with salt and pepper and place on the hot pan with the skin side up.
3. Sear the fish for 3 minutes on the other side. Set aside.
4. Using the same pan, melt the remaining butter and add the chopped pecans for about a minute. Pour the orange juice and allow to simmer for 2 minutes.

5.   Orange pecan sauce over the fish and
        sprinkle with the orange zest and
        chopped parsley. Serve.

Nutritional Values
- Calories: 350 kcal
- Fat: 33.01g
- Carbohydrates: 5.66g 65%)
- Protein: 10.87g
- Dietary Fiber : 2.8g
- Cholesterol: 38mg

Grilled Fish

(Prep Time: 35 MIN| Serve: 2)

Ingredients

- 1 lb. tilapia fillets
- 2 limes, juiced
- 1 tbsp. fresh parsley, chopped
- 1 tsp. dill
- ¼ tsp. smoked paprika
- A pinch of salt and pepper to taste
- 2 tbsp. butter

Directions

1. Place a fillet on top of one heavy duty foil.
2. Melt the butter in a saucepan heated over low fire. Pour the lemon juice, add the dill, parsley, salt and pepper.
3. Equally pour the butter on top of the fillets and season with paprika on top.
4. Wrap the fillets with the foil making sure it's secured. Cook on the grill for 5 minutes on each side.
5. Serve.

Nutritional Values
- Calories: 171 kcal
- Fat: 7.7g
- Carbohydrates: 3.06g
- Protein: 23.2g
- Dietary Fiber : 0.3g
- Cholesterol: 72mg

Buttered Shrimp

(Prep Time: 35 MIN| Serve: 2)

Ingredients

- 1 ½ lb. shrimp, peel and veins removed
- 2 tbsp. plus 6 tbsp. butter
- 4 cloves of garlic, minced
- 1 juice of lemon
- ¼ cup low-sodium chicken stock
- A pinch of salt and pepper
- 2 tbsp. fresh parsley, chopped

Directions

1. Place a skillet over medium fire and melt the butter.
2. Add the shrimps and season with salt and pepper. Stir and cook for about 3 minutes or until the shrimps turn pink. Set aside.
3. Using the same pan, sauté the garlic for 1 minute. Pour the chicken stock and juice of lemon and allow to simmer for 3-5 minutes.
4. Add the 6 tbsp. butter on to the pan and stir until it fully melts.

5.	Add the shrimp back to the pan and toss to coat with the garlic butter sauce.
6.	Garnish with chopped parsley on top before serving.

Nutritional Values

- Calories: 236 kcal
- Fat: 25.52
- Carbohydrates: 3.2g
- Protein: 35.79g
- Dietary Fiber : 0.3g
- Cholesterol: 490mg

Creamy Shrimp And Bacon Bowl

(Prep Time: 35 MIN| Serve: 2)

Ingredients

- ¼ lb. shrimps, peel and vein removed
- ¼ lb. smoked salmon, roughly chopped
- 4 bacon strips, roughly chopped
- 1 cup button mushrooms, sliced
- ½ cup coconut cream
- A pinch of salt and pepper

Directions

1. Cook the chopped bacon on a cast iron skillet over medium fire.
2. Add the sliced mushrooms when the bacon is almost crispy and then cook for another 5 minutes. Remember to stir constantly.
3. Add the salmon to the pan and cook for 2 minutes.
4. Then, add the deveined shrimp and allow to cook for another 2 minutes.
5. Pour the coconut cream on the pan and then set the heat to low fire. Allow to simmer for a minute.
6. Serve.

Nutritional Values

- Calories: 340 kcal
- Fat: 29g (86.5%)
- Carbohydrates: 3.5g
- Protein: 17g (4.5%)
- Dietary Fiber : 1g

Baked Sardines

(Prep Time: 35 MIN| Serve: 2)

Ingredients

- 800g sardines
- 1 tsp. kosher salt
- A pinch of black pepper
- 8 tbsp. extra virgin olive oil
- 4 tbsp. mint leaves, chopped
- 4 tsp. dried basil

Directions

1. Set the oven at 350F.
2. Season sardines with salt and pepper and place on a baking rack.
3. Bake in the oven for 10 minutes.
4. When done cooking, sprinkle the sardines with the mint leaves and basil and finally, drizzle with extra virgin olive oil.

Nutritional Values

- Calories: 482 kcal

- Fat: 40g (69.1%)

- Carbohydrates: 0.20g (0.2%)
- Protein: 40.01g (30.8%)
- Dietary Fiber : 0.22g

Tuna Salad

(Prep Time: 35 MIN| Serve: 2)

Ingredients

- 1 head of romaine lettuce
- 1 can tuna
- 2 hardboiled eggs, sliced
- 2 tbsp. chives, chopped
- 2 tbsp. mayonnaise
- 1 tbsp. lime juice
- 1 tbsp. olive oil
- Pinch of salt to taste

Directions

1. Tear the lettuce and place on a serving plate.
2. In a bowl, combine the tuna, mayo, lime juice, and olive oil. Season with salt and toss to coat the fish well with the dressing.
3. Serve the tuna on top of the bed of lettuce and top with the slices of egg on top.

Nutritional Values
- Calories: 996 kcal

- Fat: 45.83g
- Carbohydrates: 25.08g
- Protein: 59.75g
- Dietary Fiber : 13.7g
- Cholesterol: 1297mg

Salmon And Avocado Omelet

(Prep Time: 35 MIN| Serve: 2)

Ingredients

- 3 whole eggs
- 50g smoked salmon
- ½ avocado, sliced
- 2 tbsp. cream cheese
- 2 tbsp. chives, chopped
- 1 tbsp. butter
- A pinch of salt and pepper to taste

Directions

1. Whisk the eggs in a bowl and season with salt and pepper.
2. In a separate bowl, combine the cream cheese and chives together. Set aside.
3. Melt the butter in a non-stick pan over medium heat. Pour the egg and move the pan side to side. Cook until done.
4. Transfer the cooked egg into a plate and spread the cream cheese and chive mixture on top.

5.   Add the smoked salmon on top along with the avocado slices. Fold to create an omelet.
6.   Serve.

Nutritional Values
- Calories: 765 kcal
- Fat: 66.9g
- Carbohydrates: 13.3g
- Protein: 36.9g
- Dietary Fiber : 7.4g

Slow Cooked Lobster Bisque

(Prep Time: 35 MIN| Serve: 3)

Ingredients

- 4 pcs. lobster tails
- 1 clove of garlic
- 2 pcs. shallots, minced
- ¼ cup fresh parsley leaves, chopped
- 1 tsp. dill
- ½ tsp. smoked paprika
- ¼ tsp. ground pepper
- 2 cups heavy cream
- 4 cups low-sodium chicken broth
- 1 can diced tomatoes (with juice)

Directions

1. Place the minced garlic and shallot in a bowl and microwave on high for 2 minutes.
2. Transfer into a slow cooker and then add the rest of the ingredients except for the lobster tails and heavy cream.

3. Cut the end of the lobster tail and then add to the crockpot. Cook on high for 3 hours.

4. When done cooking, remove the lobster tails from the pot and use an immersion blender to puree the soup. This depends on the consistency you prefer your bisque to be.

5. Add the lobster back into the pot and cook for another 45 minutes.

6. Remove again the lobster and chop.

7. Pour the heavy cream into the pot along with the chopped lobster. Stir well and serve hot.

Nutritional Values

- Calories: 505 kcal
- Fat: 24.96g
- Carbohydrates: 7.12g
- Protein: 31.44g
- Dietary Fiber: 1.2g
- Cholesterol: 273mg

4.   Meats

Beefy Tacos

(Prep Time: 25 MIN| Serve: 2)

Ingredients

- 1 lb. ground beef
- 2 tbsp. butter
- 3 cloves of garlic, minced
- 1 small onion, chopped
- 1 small can of green chilies
- 1 tsp. coriander, ground
- 2 tsp. chili powder
- ½ cups sour cream
- 2 cups cheddar cheese, grated
- Lettuce cups for the wrap

Directions

1. Melt the butter in a pan over medium fire and then sauté the onion and garlic until soft.
2. Add the ground beef and then cook until done.

3. Add the green chilies, coriander and chili powder. Mix well and allow to cook for 5 minutes.

4. Turn the heat to low and then add the sour cream and cheddar. Cook for another 15 minutes.

5. Scoop the prepared taco filling into lettuce cups and serve.

Nutritional Values

- Calories: 475 kcal

- Fat: 29.97g

- Carbohydrates: 14.22g

- Protein: 36.47g

- Dietary Fiber : 0.8g

- Cholesterol: 135mg

Beef Stir-Fry

(Prep Time: 20 MIN| Serve: 2)

Ingredients

- 1 ¼ lb. ground beef
- 1 tbsp. clarified butter
- 3 cloves of garlic
- ¼ tsp. ginger, minced
- 1 tsp. red pepper flakes
- ¼ cup coconut aminos
- ½ tsp. liquid stevia
- ½ tsp. molasses
- 2 pcs. green onions, chopped

Directions

1. Place a wok or skillet over medium fire. Melt the butter and then add the ground beef. Cook for a few minutes until brown.
2. Add the liquid stevia, coconut aminos, molasses and red pepper flakes and then stir and allow to simmer for 3-4 minutes.
3. Garnish with chopped green onions on top before serving.

Nutritional Values

- Calories: 324 kcal
- Fat: 20.93g
- Carbohydrates: 3.28g
- Protein: 29.15g
- Dietary Fiber : 0.7g
- Cholesterol: 106mg

Beef Balls In Creamy Sauce

(Prep Time: 15 MIN| Serve: 3)

Ingredients

- 1 ½ lb. ground beef
- 2 tbsp. Worcestershire sauce
- 3 tbsp. fresh parsley, chopped
- 3 cloves of garlic, minced
- 1 tsp. garlic powder
- 1 small onion, diced
- 1 tsp. onion powder
- Salt and pepper to taste
- 2 tbsp. clarified butter
- 2 tbsp. butter
- ½ cup sliced button mushrooms
- 1 cup low-sodium beef stock
- 2 tbsp. cooking sherry
- 2 tbsp. beef bouillon granules
- ¼ cup heavy cream
- ¾ cup sour cream

Directions

1. In a large bowl, mix together the ground beef, one clove of the minced garlic, chopped parsley, Worcestershire, garlic powder

and onion powder. Season with salt and pepper. Combine the ingredients with your hands and then create 4 patties.

2. Heat the clarified butter in a pan over medium-high fire. Place the patties and sear for about 2 minutes on each side. Remove the patties and set aside.

3. Using the same pan, melt the butter and drizzle the cooking sherry. Lower the fire and add the diced onion, button mushrooms, and the rest of the minced garlic. Cook until the onions are caramelized.

4. Pour the beef stock into the pan and also add the bouillon granules.

5. Add the heavy cream and sour cream into the pan, followed by the browned patties. Allow to simmer on low fire for 10 minutes. Serve.

Nutritional Values

- Calories: 714 kcal

- Fat: 48.49g

- Carbohydrates: 19.73g
- Protein: 49.25g
- Dietary Fiber : 1.1g
- Cholesterol: 210mg

Beefy, Gooey Cheese, Goodness

(Prep Time: 35 MIN| Serve: 2)

Ingredients

- 1 lb. ground beef
- 1 cup cheddar cheese, grated
- 1 cup baby spinach, chopped
- 1 small bell pepper, chopped
- 5 free-range eggs
- A dash of salt and pepper to taste

Directions

1. Set the oven at 350F.
2. Place the ground beef on a skillet and cook until brown.
3. Transfer the cooked beef on a mixing bowl and then add the baby spinach and red pepper. Combine well.
4. Place the beef and spinach mixture into a baking dish greased with butter making sure it is well distributed onto the dish.
5. On another bowl, whisk the eggs and season with salt and pepper.

6. Add the cheddar cheese on top of the beef and then followed by the whisked egg.
7. Place the in the oven to bake for 18-20 minutes. Allow to cool for a few minutes before cutting into squares and serving.

Nutritional Values

- Calories: 391 kcal

- Fat: 22.41g

- Carbohydrates: 7.61g

- Protein: 40.85g

- Dietary Fiber : 1.4g

- Cholesterol: 333mg

Beef Sausage And Bacon Pot

(Prep Time: 15 MIN| Serve: 2)

Ingredients

- 1 lb. beef sausage
- 8 pcs. bacon strips, chopped
- 2 cups broccoli florets
- ½ cup heavy cream
- 1 tbsp. Dijon mustard
- ¼ cup cheddar cheese, grated

Directions

1. Set oven at 350F.
2. Cut the sausages into chunks and place on a baking dish with the chopped bacon.
3. Also add the florets into the dish making sure they're equally distributed.
4. In a small bowl, combine the cream and mustard and pour on top of the meat and broccoli.
5. Finally, sprinkle the top of the dish with the grated cheese and bake in the oven for 35 minutes.
6. Serve.

Nutritional Values

- Calories: 768 kcal
- Fat: 58.96g
- Carbohydrates: 5.58g
- Protein: 46.81g
- Dietary Fiber : 8.3g
- Cholesterol: 42mg

Filet Mignon Steak

(Prep Time: 20 MIN| Serve: 2)

Ingredients

- 2 large (about 1.5 inch thick) filet mignon steaks, cut in half
- 2 tbsp. ghee
- A pinch of salt and pepper to taste

Directions

1. Set oven at 275F
2. Take a paper towel and pat dry the steaks and then season with salt and pepper.
3. Lay the steaks on a baking rack on top of a baking sheet lined with foil.
4. Place in the oven to broil for 30 minutes or until the meat registers at 90F.
5. Remove the steaks from the oven and then place on a skillet with ghee over high heat.
6. Cook the steaks for about 2 minutes on each side.

7. Reduce the heat to medium and then brown all sides for another 1 minute each.
8. Serve with your favorite steak sauce.

Nutritional Values

- Calories: 22 kcal

- Fat: 15.85g

- Carbohydrates: 1.06g

- Protein: 17.77g

- Dietary Fiber : 0.2g

- Cholesterol: 75mg

Curried Ground Beef

(Prep Time: 25 MIN| Serve: 2)

Ingredients

- 1 lb. ground beef
- 3 pcs. carrots, chopped
- 1 pc. large tomato, chopped
- 1 tsp. mustard seeds
- 1 onion, chopped
- A handful of curry leaves
- 4 cloves of garlic, minced
- ½ tsp. ginger, minced
- 1 tsp. coriander powder
- ¼ tsp. chili powder
- ½ tsp. turmeric
- ½ tsp. sea salt
- 2 tsp. masala
- 2 tbsp. ghee
- 1 can coconut milk
- ¼ cup water

Directions

1. Heat the ghee on a pan over medium fire.

2. Throw in the mustard seeds and wait until the seeds start to pop before adding the chopped onion and curry leaves.
3. Sauté for 3 minutes and then add the minced garlic and ginger. Stir and then add the rest of the spices.
4. Add the ground beef and cook until brown.
5. Add the chopped potato and carrots and pour the ¼ cup water. Cover and simmer for 5 minutes.
6. Pour in the coconut milk, stir and cook for 15 minutes, or until the veggies are soft.
7. Serve.

Nutritional Values

- Calories: 332 kcal

- Fat: 19.1g

- Carbohydrates: 13.9g

- Protein: 30.g

- Dietary Fiber : 3.1g

- Cholesterol: 100mg

5.   Veggies

Roast Peppers with Zucchini

(Prep Time: 15 MIN| Serve: 2)

Ingredients

- 2 bell peppers, cut in chunks
- 3 zucchini, cut in chunks
- ½ cup garlic cloves, peeled
- Seasoning: salt, pepper, Italian seasoning to taste
- 2 tbsp. olive oil

Directions

1. Add the vegetables and oil to a greased crockpot. Season with salt, pepper and Italian seasoning.
2. Close the lid. Cook for 3 hours on high.

Nutritional Values

- Calories: 97kcal
- Fat: 7.4 g
- Carbohydrates: 7.7g
- Protein: 2.3g
- Dietary Fiber : 7g
- Cholesterol: 24mg

Tomatoes, Asparagus & Squash

(Prep Time: 10 MIN| Serve: 2)

Ingredients

- 15 oz tomatoes, diced
- 10 oz asparagus, cut in large pieces
- 10 oz summer squash, cut in large pieces
- 10 oz marrow squash, cut in large pieces
- Seasoning: salt, pepper, garlic, onion powder, basil to taste

Directions

1. Add diced tomatoes to the bottom of a crockpot.
2. On top of tomatoes, place the vegetables. Season with salt, pepper and herbs.
3. Close the lid. Cook for 3 hours on high.

Nutritional Values

- Calories: 38 kcal

- Fat: 0.4
- Carbohydrates: 9g
- Protein: 3g
- Dietary Fiber : 3.1g
- Cholesterol: 0mg

Cheesy Cauliflower with Mushrooms

(Prep Time: 10 MIN| Serve: 2)

Ingredients

- 4 cups frozen cauliflower, thawed
- ½ cup onion, chopped
- 10 oz white mushrooms, sliced
- 2 cups American cheese, shredded
- Salt, pepper to taste

Directions

1. Combine vegetables and mushrooms with cheese in a crockpot. Season with salt and pepper.
2. Close the lid. Cook for 4 hours on low.

Nutritional Values

- Calories: 366 kcal

- Fat: 22g

- Carbohydrates: 18g

- Protein: 25.g

- Dietary Fiber : 2.3g

- Cholesterol: 0mg

Eggplant Parmigiana

(Prep Time: 6 MIN| Serve: 2)

Ingredients

- 3 medium eggplants, peeled, cut in 2 inch slices
- 1/3 cup seasoned bread crumbs
- ½ cup Parmesan, grated
- 32 oz marinara sauce
- Salt, pepper to taste

Directions

1. Using olive oil, sauté the eggplants in a large skillet until lightly brown.
2. In a separate bowl combine the seasoned bread crumbs with grated Parmesan.
3. Layer the eggplants into a crockpot beginning with eggpland, next top with crumbs, then marinara sauce. Repeat layers.
4. Close the lid and cook for 5 hours on low.

Nutritional Values

- Calories: 353 kcal

- Fat: 13g

- Carbohydrates: 51g

- Protein: 13g

- Dietary Fiber : 3.1g

- Cholesterol: 0mg

Glazed Carrots

(Prep Time: 5 MIN| Serve: 2)

Ingredients

- 2 lb baby carrots, washed
- 3 tbsp. maple syrup
- 2 tbsp. coconut oil
- ¼ cup water
- Salt, herbs (rosemary, thyme, dill) to taste

Directions

1. Add all ingredients into a crockpot bowl.
2. Close the lid and cook for 5 hours on high. Stir the carrots after 4 hours cooking.

Nutritional Values

- Calories: 70 kcal

- Fat: 1.3g

- Carbohydrates: 14.5g

- Protein: 0.8g

- Dietary Fiber : 3.1g

- Cholesterol: 0mg

Turnip Greens

(Prep Time: 5 MIN| Serve: 2)

Ingredients

- 3 turnips, peeled, quartered
- 2 bunches fresh turnip greens, washed, chopped
- ½ lb ham hock
- 1 pinch red pepper flakes
- 1 cup water

Directions

1. Add half of greens to a crockpot with 1 cup of water. Add the turnips, ham hock and red pepper.
2. Close the lid and cook for 1 hour on low. Then add the remaining greens.
3. Cook for 6 hours on low.

Nutritional Values

- Calories: 114 kcal

- Fat: 6.7g

- Carbohydrates: 5g

- Protein: 8.6g

- Dietary Fiber : 3.1g

- Cholesterol: 0mg

Bacon-flavored Cabbage

(Prep Time: 5 MIN| Serve: 2)

Ingredients

- 1 small head of cabbage, cored, chopped
- 2/3 cup cooked, crumbled bacon
- 15 oz pearl onions,
- 8 cups chicken broth
- Salt, pepper to taste

Directions

1. Place the chopped cabbage into a crockpot.
2. Top with onions and bacon. Season with salt and pepper.
3. Pour the broth over the cabbage.
4. Close the lid and cook for 6 hours on high.

Nutritional Values

- Calories: 138 kcal

- Fat: 6g

- Carbohydrates: 11.5g

- Protein: 9g

- Dietary Fiber : 3.1g

- Cholesterol: 0mg

Yellow Squash Casserole

(Prep Time: 5 MIN| Serve: 2)

Ingredients

- 2 lb yellow squash, sliced across
- 1 cup chopped onion
- 2 cups salted crackers , crumbled
- 1 cup Cheddar cheese, shredded
- 1 tbsp. butter

Directions

1. Microwave squash, onion and 1 tablespoon butter for 10 minutes uncovered.
2. Add the squash mixture together with ½ cup cheese and 1 cup cracker crumbs into a crockpot.
3. In a separate bowl combine the remaining cheese with 1 cup of cracker crumbs, and sprinkle over the squash.
4. Close the lid and cook for 2 hours on low.
5. Turn the heat off and let stand for 30 min

Nutritional Values

- Calories: 97 kcal

- Fat: 5g

- Carbohydrates: 6g

- Protein: 5g

- Dietary Fiber : 3.1g

- Cholesterol: 0mg

Roasted Zucchini with Onion

(Prep Time: 5 MIN| Serve: 2)

Ingredients

- 2 carrots, peeled, sliced
- ½ onion, sliced
- 2 zucchini, cubed thickly
- 2 tbsp. olive oil
- 1 packet Italian dressing mix, dry

Directions

1. Place the vegetables into a crockpot bowl. Sprinkle with oil and Italian seasoning. Toss well.
2. Close the lid and cook for 6 hours on low.
3. Serve with Parmesan cheese if desired.

Nutritional Values

- Calories: 410 kcal

- Fat: 3.5g

- Carbohydrates: 2.6g

- Protein: 0.3g

- Dietary Fiber : 3.1g

- Cholesterol: 0mg

6. Desserts

Keto Peanut Butter Popsicles

(Prep Time: 15 MIN| Serve: 2)

Ingredients

- 1 cup peanut butter
- ½ vanilla extract
- 1 cup whipping cream
- ¼ cup granulated sugar
- ¼ cup swerve
- 8 oz. cream cheese
- 4 oz. baking unsweetened chocolate
- 4 pkts Stevia

Directions

1. Mix the peanut butter, vanilla extract, whipping cream, granulated sugar, swerve, cream cheese together.
2. Spoon the mixture into popsicle molds
3. Place a popsicle stick into each mold.
4. Freeze 6 hours or overnight
5. Remove the popsicles by running the mold under hot water.
6. Melt the baking chocolate and add Stevia.

7.	Dip the popsicle in the chocolate.
8.	Place the dipped popsicles on a parchment paper to cool.
9.	Place the dipped popsicles in freezer.
10.	Serve it.

Nutritional Values

- Calories: 203kcal
- Fat: 18g
- Carbohydrates: 11g
- Protein: 5g
- Dietary Fiber : 7g
- Cholesterol: 24mg

Yummy Brownies

(Prep Time: 15 MIN| Serve: 2)

Ingredients

Brownies
- ¾ cup granulated erythritol
- ½ cup coconut flour
- ½ cup butter ghee
- 2 tbsp cocoa powder
- 3 eggs
- 1tsp baking soda
- ½ cup brewed organic coffee
- 6 tbsp. unsweetened almond milk
- 1¼ tsp apple cider vinegar
- 1 tsp vanilla extract

Frosting
- ¼ coconut oil
- 1½ tbsp unsweetened almond milk
- ½ tsp organic vanilla extract
- ½ cup erythritol
- 1 tbsp cocoa powder

Directions

1. Preheat oven at 400F
2. Oil the pan well

3.   Mix the coconut flour and erythritol together in a bowl. Set aside.
4.   Mix butter ghee with brewed coffee and cocoa powder. Stir and heat to boiling on stove top.
5.   Combine both mix and Stir well.
6.   Add 3 eggs, almond milk, baking soda, vanilla extract and apple cider vinegar mixture into the combined mixture.
7.   Use an electric mixer to mix them together.
8.   Pour the mixture into the pan.
9.   Bake at 400F for 20 minutes
10.   Prepare the frosting by mixing the butter ghee, almond milk and cocoa powder in a saucepan.
11.   Stir and heat to a boil. Change to lowest heat.
12.   Add erythritol and vanilla extract. Stir well. Maintain lowest heat.
13.   Pour warm frosting over the brownies. Use spoon to spread.
14.   Cool brownies and frosting.
15.   Place it in the fridge for further cooling. Approx. 1 hour.
16.   Slice and Serve it.

Nutritional Values

- Calories: 171kcal
- Fat: 16g
- Carbohydrates: 2g

- Protein: 3g
- Dietary Fiber : 2.2g
- Cholesterol: 0 mg

Keto Lemon Curd

(Prep Time: 10 MIN| Serve: 2)

Ingredients

- 2 organic eggs
- 2 organic egg yolks
- 3tbsp. granulated erythritol
- 6 tbsp. butter cubes
- ½ cup organic lemon juice

Directions

1. Mix the lemon juice, erythritol, egg and egg yolks together in a pan.
2. Add the butter cubes and turn on the stove and adjust to lowest heat
3. Stir well
4. Once the butter melts, turn the heat up to medium-high
5. Stir until thicken.
6. Pour the mix over a sieve or mesh strainer to remove any egg bits.
7. Place it in fridge.

Nutritional Values

- Calories: 200kcal
- Fat: 20g
- Carbohydrates: 1g
- Protein: 3g
- Dietary Fiber : 0g
- Cholesterol: 60mg

Low Carb Cheesecake Brownie

(Prep Time: 30 MIN| Serve: 2)

Ingredients

Cheesecake Filling
- 2 eggs
- ¼ cup heavy cream
- ½ cup granulated erythritol
- ½ tsp vanilla extract
- 1 lb cream cheese, softened

Brownie
- 2 eggs
- ¼ cup cocoa powder
- pinch sea salt
- ¼ cup chopped walnuts
- ¼ tsp vanilla
- ¾ cup granulated erythritol
- ½ cup butter
- 2 oz. unsweetened chocolate
- ½ cup almond flour

Directions

1. Preheat oven to 325F
2. Butter the sauce pan and wrap the bottom with foil

3. Melt butter and chocolate in the microwave oven in 30 seconds interval until smooth.
4. Mix the sea salt, almond flour and cocoa powder in a small bowl.
5. Beat eggs with erythritol and vanilla until smooth in a bowl.
6. Add the almond flour and beat it
7. Add the butter chocolate mixture and beat it till smooth.
8. Stir well
9. Spread evenly over bottom of prepared pan.
10. Bake 15 to 20 minutes until it is soft in the center.
11. Set aside to cool for 20 minutes
12. For Cheesecake filling, reduce to 300F
13. Beat cream cheese until smooth.
14. Beat eggs with erythritol and vanilla until smooth in a bowl.
15. Pour filling over crust and place the cheesecake on a bake sheet.
16. Bake until edges are set and center is soft. Approx. 35 – 45 minutes.
17. Remove from oven and cool down.
18. Loosen the edge with knife.
19. Cover with plastic wrap and refrigerate for 3 hours.
20. Serve it.

Nutritional Values

- Calories: 381 kcal
- Fat: 34g
- Carbohydrates: 7g
- Protein: 9g
- Dietary Fiber : 2g
- Cholesterol: 156mg

Coconut Oil Candies

(Prep Time: 25 MIN| Serve: 2)

Ingredients

- 4 tbsp unsweetened cocoa powder
- 1 cup softened cold pressed coconut oil
- 1 tbsp. swerve
- 1 tbsp. vanilla extract
- ½ tsp sea salt
- 3 tbsp. organic unsweetened cocoa powder

Directions

1. Combine the ingredients in a bowl
2. Mix until smooth
3. Drop by tablespoon onto a parchment paper
4. Refrigerate until candies solidify.
5. Store in a covered container in the fridge.

Nutritional Values

- Calories: 76 kcal
- Fat: 8g
- Carbohydrates: 2.45g
- Protein: 1g
- Dietary Fiber : 1g

- Cholesterol: 73mg

Mint Fudge

(Prep Time: 20 MIN| Serve: 2)

Ingredients

- 2 tbsp. vanilla extract
- 1 tsp peppermint extract
- 1½ cup pumpkin seeds
- ½ cup dried parsley flakes
- 1 cup cold pressed coconut oil
- ¼ tbsp. sea salt
- ½ cup of swerve

Directions

- Melt coconut oil in saucepan.
- Add all ingredients into blender, follow by the warm coconut oil and blend until smooth.
- Pour into a baking pan.
- Freeze it for 4 hours.
- Retrieve and cut into pieces.
- Store in refrigerator to prevent softening.

Nutritional Values
- Calories: 119kcal

- Fat: 9g (66.9%)
- Carbohydrates: 9.5g (19.8%)
- Protein: 4g (13.2%)
- Dietary Fiber : 3.5g
- Cholesterol: 0 mg

Keto Avocado Pudding

(Prep Time: 5 MIN| Serve: 2)

Ingredients

- 2 avocados
- 1 tbsp. fresh lime juice
- 400ml organic coconut milk
- 2 tsp organic vanilla extract
- 80 drops stevia
- 1 tbsp. Cacao Nibs

Directions

- Peeled, pitted and slice the avocado into pieces
- Add the ingredients into a blender
- Blend until smooth. Sprinkle cacao nibs on top.
- Serve it.

Nutritional Values

- Calories: 292kcal
- Fat: 28.8g
- Carbohydrates: 3.8g
- Protein: 2.7g
- Dietary Fiber : 0g
- Cholesterol: 0mg

Coconut Pudding

(Prep Time: 7 MIN| Serve: 2)

Ingredients

- 1½ coconut milk
- 1 tbsp. beef gelatin
- 3 egg yolks
- ½ tsp vanilla extract
- 6 tbsp. stevia

Directions

1. Mix the gelatin and 1 tbsp. coconut milk in a small bowl. Set aside.
2. Heat the saucepan and add the remaining coconut milk and stevia.
3. Stir for 3 -5 minutes.
4. Pour the hot coconut milk over the egg yolks and whisk it continuously.
5. Transfer the hot mixture back into a pot and cook for 3 – 4 minutes until thicken.
6. Pour the small bowl of gelatin into the pot and stir well.
7. Pour the mixture evenly into 2 ramekins.
8. Refrigerate it for 3 hours to set it
9. Serve it.

Nutritional Values
- Calories: 291kcal
- Fat: 8.8g
- Carbohydrates: 45g
- Protein: 7.6g
- Dietary Fiber : 1.8g
- Cholesterol: 15mg

Conclusion

I hope that by the end of reading this book: Ketogenic Diet, that you'll see that this is true, and that a Ketogenic is available to anyone and everyone. It's very affordable, it's good wholesome food, it's nothing complicated, you don't require any specialist equipment, there's nothing faddy about the diet; instead it's straightforward common sense, of cutting out carbohydrates and eating more fat. Some people are under the impression that meat is expensive and that they simply can't afford to eat it very often, and therefore think that a ketogenic/low-carbohydrate diet wouldn't be accessible to them. We're not however talking about expensive joints of meat that you need to purchase. Many of the recipes include chicken, bacon, turkey, ham, minced beef, all of which you can pick up inexpensively, and because these are the core bits to your diet, and you're no longer purchasing processed foods or carbohydrates, you will see no difference to the cost of your shopping bills.

This diet is perfect if you're wanting to lose weight and improve your health. This book has explained all about a ketogenic diet and the balance of food, and the types of food you need to eat, in order to achieve the state of ketosis. It also mentions the types of food that you should avoid. By eating a Ketogenic diet, there are so many benefits for your health too. Not only will you lose weight, but your cholesterol will improve, your blood sugar and blood pressure will reduce, and there's a wealth of other conditions/diseases that by eating a Ketogenic diet, you're at less risk of contracting.

This book, also gives you a diet plan template for a week, of the types of food that you 'could' choose to eat for breakfast, lunch and tea; and there are 12 recipes at the end of the book. 6 of these recipes are ones which you can make using just 5 key ingredients or less, which demonstrates the simplicity and low-cost factor of this diet.

This book has hopefully shown you that you don't need to eat less; you just learn to eat smarter food options, much less carbohydrates (only about 5%) and much greater fats (about 75%). You'll have learned the sensible rate that you should ideally be losing weight at. You'll have learned about the foods that you can, and can't eat (it's mostly just carbohydrates that are the key restriction). There are foods however, that are more sensible options, that will make you feel fuller for longer. You'll have learned how the Body Mass Index (BMI) is calculated, and how you work out approximately where your BMI is, but also to take into account

that this isn't set in stone, just an approximate
guide. By losing 10% of your body weight, this can
have a dramatic positive impact.